AF394081

INCREASE YOUR SELF-ESTEEM

Learn to be happy in your own skin

Written by Irène Guittin
Translated by Rebecca Neal

Health and Wellbeing · 50MINUTES.com

INCREASE YOUR SELF-ESTEEM

- **Problem:** we have all felt self-conscious about something at one point or another. Whether we have a body part we do not like, an inferiority complex or even a surname that we find embarrassing, these insidious hang-ups can soon have a negative impact on our personal, professional or social lives if we are unable to move past them.
- **Aims:** to start viewing your insecurities positively and feel more comfortable in your own skin.
- **FAQs:**
  - Are we all equally susceptible to feeling self-conscious?
  - Are our insecurities caused by the media?
  - Although I am well into adulthood, my mother's criticisms still affect me. Is this normal?
  - Is psychoanalysis necessary to improve my self-esteem?

- I have tried everything to feel good about my body, but it still disgusts me. Is cosmetic surgery the only solution?
- I feel unsophisticated compared to other people. How can I hide this from them?
- My colleagues make fun of my lack of character. How can I start standing up for myself?
- My friends make fun of my lisp. How can I tell them that I find their jokes hurtful?

All of us, no matter our background, have things that we feel self-conscious about, but these things are typically difficult to pin down, understand and overcome. They are complex and contradictory: they are at once universal and taboo, shared and intimate, tangible and concealed, and they both help shape our identity and hold us back. Although all of us will struggle with insecurities at one point or another, we can control how much we let them affect us and how we deal with them.

Insecurities are generally thought of as the enemy, and this can be clearly seen in the language we use to talk about them: we talk about beating or overcoming them, terms which suggest a battle or struggle which can only end when we destroy our opponent or they destroy us.

Although insecurities are often viewed as external threats that can be destroyed, in reality they are a part of us and play a role in our personal development. This is both normal and unavoidable; the important thing is therefore to not let ourselves be beaten down, but rather to control, accept and even appreciate the things we feel most self-conscious about. Conversely, if we let ourselves fixate on them, our daily lives and relationships with other people will suffer. Putting time and effort into working on our self-esteem is therefore essential, as our wellbeing depends on self-acceptance.

INSECURITIES: THE ENEMY WITHIN

WHERE DO OUR INSECURITIES COME FROM?

The role of the past

Psychologists unanimously accept that our insecurities have multiple causes, but that these causes generally come from within the person themselves (their experiences and personality) and the environment they grew up in (their upbringing and schooling). You should therefore find that many of your current problems can be explained by your past.

Life stages

Our tendency to fixate on imperfections, which can be physical or mental and real or imagined, most often emerges at pivotal moments in our lives, such as adolescence, the start of adulthood or during a mid-life crisis, as these periods are important as we search for and build our identities. It is also possible to develop a complex after a particular event which makes us feel insecure and doubt ourselves, whether or not the reasons for this are rational. For example, even naturally confident people may fall apart after losing their job ("I've been fired because I can't talk to people, I'm useless") or going through a difficult break-up ("She left me because I'm boring", "He broke up with me because I got fat").

Social pressure

Our self-esteem is influenced not only by our experiences, but also by the people around us. Our parents, who are the earliest influences we come into contact with and help shape us as people, can often leave us feeling self-conscious and insecure, generally without realising it. Many parents want the best for their children, which leads them to be very demanding: while their aim is to push their child towards excellence, they may not realise that the child feels demoralised and as though they will never live up to their parents' expectations.

Cutting remarks

We have all made or been on the receiving end of comments that seem harmless, but that can cut deep: "It's not hard to understand, are you stupid or are you doing it on purpose?", "No man would want you, you can't do anything right", "It's time for you to get to the gym", "What are we going to do with you?", and so on. People may make these kinds of comments without giving them a second thought, but they can severely dent the self-esteem of sensitive people. Our classmates at school also often plant the seeds of future insecurities, as playground taunts can have a lasting impact. Children can be cruel, and will not think twice about laughing at an unusual surname, braces, a particular hair colour or a person's size. However, these taunts can leave invisible scars that stay with their victims well into adulthood.

WHAT ARE THE DIFFERENT TYPES OF INSECURITIES?

Physical insecurities

In our society, appearances play a decisive role in our impressions of a person or thing, which explains why we can develop deep-rooted insecurities over the slightest physical quirk. Whether we are flat-chested or on the curvy side, thin-lipped or fuller-lipped, very thin or a bit larger, thick-haired or balding, we can struggle with the fact that we do not match some arbitrary "ideal".

Mental insecurities

The fact that mental insecurities are often better-hidden and less immediately obvious than physical insecurities does not mean that they are any less common or difficult to deal with. Even though nobody is perfect, we often struggle in certain areas and feel inferior because we cannot do mental maths or because we know nothing about medieval history, philosophy, mechanics, fashion or DIY.

Insecurities due to our environment

Our lifestyle and upbringing can also give rise to insecurities. Inferiority complexes can affect both people who grew up in unstable environments (as they fear being rejected because of their reputation) and those who had a more privileged upbringing (as they fear that they will be seen as snobbish or that their successes will be chalked up to their background rather than their own merits). Similarly, inferiority complexes can strike both mollycoddled only children (as they never learn to stand on their own two feet) and children with many siblings (as they are given less attention). In all families, backgrounds and groups, there are factors that can contribute to low self-esteem.

WHAT ROLE DOES THE MEDIA PLAY?

The media is often accused of playing a major role in self-esteem problems. It is true that it places a lot of importance on appearance, success and happiness and sets unattainable standards, but it would not be fair to say that it is the cause of the problem. Rather, it exacerbates or reveals the true extent of our insecurities, as self-esteem issues come from within us.

It is nonetheless undeniable that the media aggravates and fuels our insecurities. The toned, slender physiques we see in advertisements, the success stories that appear on the news and the heroes of Hollywood films are far removed from most people's daily lives, but this does not stop us from comparing ourselves to these largely fictional personas: we want Will Smith's muscles, Victoria Beckham's slim figure, Steve Jobs's creativity, Kate Middleton's elegance, Bill Gates's wealth, and so on. The media encourages us in this, as celebrity magazines and television programmes peddle these images and portray them as the ultimate goal if we want to be happy and successful.

DID YOU KNOW?

The images on magazine covers are generally retouched to eliminate any perceived imperfections and give the illusion of "perfection", as dictated by society's beauty standards. For example, any blemishes will be erased, the model or celebrity may be made thinner, their eyes will be brightened, and so on, which means that the stars on magazine covers are really not all that different from the rest of us.

It is pointless, and possibly even dangerous, to view celebrities as role models. We are all different, in terms of our experiences, environment, physique and personality. Remember that the media never shows us the full picture, and that it manipulates images and facts to make them conform to particular ideals and standards.

WHY ARE INSECURITIES SO DIFFICULT TO GET RID OF?

The reason that insecurities are so dangerous and harmful is that they are self-perpetuating. Their root cause is an inability to view ourselves correctly and objectively: it is not the individual who is flawed, but rather their self-image, and this distorts everything they see. They fixate on illusions until they believe that they are reality, and these illusions can soon become obsessions if they are not careful. When somebody regularly or constantly puts themselves down, they end up convincing themselves and other people that their flaws are real. However, there is some good news: becoming aware of the danger is the first step towards breaking this vicious circle.

BODY DYSMORPHIC DISORDER

Body dysmorphic disorder (BDD) is characterised by an individual's obsessive belief that one or more parts of their body are deformed or imperfect. It is the pathological form of physical insecurities and can lead to the individual becoming withdrawn or even developing social phobia. In some cases, the sufferer is so disgusted by their own body that every waking moment is torture. In this case, therapy is vital, as BDD can also lead to extreme behaviour intended to control or eliminate the perceived faults, such as eating disorders or a reliance on cosmetic surgery. This illness should not be taken lightly, as it can cause irreversible physical and mental damage if it is left untreated.

A DAILY STRUGGLE

HOW CAN YOU FIGHT YOUR DEMONS?

The first step in winning the battle is to break the vicious circle which fuels and exacerbates your insecurities. This involves breaking your old habits, fighting your natural instinct to put yourself down and ignoring the little voice in your head that tells you that you are worthless. Whatever you may think, these harmful, negative thoughts do not reflect who you really are.

Keep paranoia in check

Do not let yourself become isolated or cut yourself off from the world and your friends and family because of your self-esteem issues. Do not be afraid to take risks and open up to other people without immediately thinking that they wish you harm or are judging you behind your back: you are your own worst critic.

People suffering from self-esteem problems generally imagine other people's reactions and feel humiliated by them. You therefore need to force yourself to think and respond positively: stop imagining that everyone is staring at your nose, as you are probably the only one who thinks it is too big; stop thinking that everyone is laughing at how unsophisticated you are, as in reality they probably appreciate your sense of humour; and do not think that everyone you meet is focusing on how short you are – they may actually be impressed by your boundless energy.

Do not let your insecurities control your life

Letting your insecurities dictate what you do will only make them worse, and it will also stop you from living your life. Enjoy every moment without dwelling on negative thoughts: go to the beach in a swimming costume even though you have put on a bit of weight; tie your hair back even though your ears stick out; do not be afraid to show your braces when you smile; and stay on the dancefloor until the end of the night even if you have no sense of rhythm.

Another common mistake is to blame all your

personal and professional failures or difficulties on your insecurities. You are the only person who can control your life, so it is up to you to accept yourself and avoid letting minor flaws throw you off course, hold you back and stop you from thriving.

Victor, 43, confesses that for a long time used his inferiority complex as an excuse for all his problems:

> "My family is working class, and for a long time I thought that the reason I struggled at school was that my parents never went to university. I was convinced that I was going to in their footsteps and never bothered thinking about my future. I was so self-conscious about my past failures that I had no professional ambition. When I was at secondary school, one of my teachers made me see that the only thing holding me back was my own self-doubt. He gave me a leg up and got me to believe in myself, and I was so motivated that I caught up. I'm now a financial director at a big company and give classes in the hope that I can pay it forward and help young people to overcome their insecurities."

Trust the people around you

As long as you let your insecurities control you, you will be unable to make progress. You need to force yourself to move past them. This will inevitably be difficult to begin with, but it is an essential step, and there is no need to go through it alone. Although improving your self-esteem is a personal journey, you should not hesitate to ask your friends and family to support you through it. Keep in mind that they want the best for you and will probably be more than happy to help you, work with you to rebuild your self-esteem and watch you thrive. Even if you do not see yourself as smart or beautiful, they do! Listen to their encouragement and compliments, accept their efforts to comfort you and take advantage of the friendly ear they offer you.

On the other hand, you do not have to stay close to people who fuel your insecurities or make you feel worse about yourself; instead, focus on your relationships with positive people who want the best for you. If you have a friend who makes digs at your body every time you go clothes shopping together, feel free to limit your contact with them. Remember that anyone who feels the need to put you down is no doubt struggling with their own self-esteem!

Put things into perspective

It is not easy to admit, but a person who fixates constantly on their perceived flaws and is convinced that everyone else's attention is riveted on them Is behaving somewhat egocentrically. Remember that other people almost certainly do not pay as much attention to the things you dislike about yourself as you do, so make sure you keep things in perspective. In the same way that you are not constantly thinking about the gap in your friend's front teeth, your colleague's slight lisp or your cousin's big feet, they are certainly not fixated on your minor flaws – or the features that you think are flaws.

In his bestselling book *The Power of Now*, Eckhart Tolle demonstrates that we are the main obstacle standing in the way of our own fulfilment: "This incessant mental noise prevents you from finding that realm of inner stillness that is inseparable from Being. It also creates a false mind-made self that casts a shadow of fear and suffering".

Learn to take a step back and put things into perspective. Everyone has their flaws, and this is what makes the world such an interesting place! Take back control of your life and accept yourself just as you are.

QUICK TIP

Many people suffering from low self-esteem are hypersensitive, at least when it comes to certain touchy subjects. Learning to take things less personally is another step towards self-acceptance and greater self-confidence. When you feel attacked and can feel your anger mounting, take a few deep breaths and try to work out why you are so hurt by what the other person has just said. Taking the time to reflect will not only give your anger time to abate, but will also allow you to put things into perspective and reason with yourself. Over time, you will stop taking throwaway remarks to heart as much and may be able to laugh at yourself instead.

Consult a specialist

If you want to overcome your insecurities, you need to not only work out where they come from, but also have the right tools at your disposal to tackle them. Some people find that seeking expert help in the form of psychoanalysis is a good way of getting to know themselves better, and of identifying and understanding the subconscious mechanisms that explain why they are anxious and why they feel and react the way that they do. As understanding is often the first step towards healing, psychoanalysis can be a good way of dealing with your insecurities on a day-to-day basis. However, it is a long process, and although the happiness and relief it can bring make it worth the effort, it can be challenging and difficult at times.

Psychoanalysis is not for everyone, and it is far from the only way of working on your self-esteem. If you are unsure, do not force yourself to do it, as this may cause your problems to become further entrenched and complicate the process. Feel free to explore as many other options as you want until you find the one that works best for you.

HOW CAN YOU OVERCOME YOUR INSECURITIES?

Accept your imperfections

The road to self-acceptance is a long one. One of the most difficult, but absolutely essential, steps, is facing up to reality. Avoiding your insecurities is not an effective long-term solution, as they will inevitably re-emerge sooner or later.

Overcoming your insecurities means facing up to them and accepting the person you see when you look in the mirror. Do not avoid your reflection; instead, look at it objectively, familiarise yourself with it and stop judging it and putting it down. You can do this by looking at it as though it were someone else: in doing so, you will see that it may not be perfect, but that its imperfections are all part of its charm and that it has plenty of good points too.

For example, if you have never been able to quieten your loud, attention-grabbing laugh, remind yourself that it shows people that you are happy and spreads joy to others. Similarly, if you feel unfeminine because you think you are too flat-chested, banish this thought from your mind and embrace plunging necklines.

Louisa, 32, let being very tall get in the way of her social life until she made it her main asset:

> "Since I was 15, I've been a head taller than everyone else. For a long time, I just wanted the ground to swallow me up and hide me. I was too afraid to talk to people, and especially to boys, as I thought that nobody could find a giant like me feminine or attractive. But that's exactly what happened! Even though Ben is shorter than me, he's never been intimidated by the height difference. He managed to make me feel feminine and give me confidence in myself. Now I even wear heels, which would have been unthinkable in the past."

Recognise your good points

As our insecurities come from a distorted, unreasonably negative self-image, it is important to force ourselves to see things positively. Focus on developing your good points – you undoubtedly have plenty of them! Rather than fixating on minor flaws, focus your attention on your physical and mental strengths and draw attention to them.

Accept compliments

It is a truism that we only hear what we want to hear. Furthermore, we hear, or rather subconsciously choose to remember, what we expect to hear. If you are convinced that the people around you do not have a good word to say about you, you will only see and hear the negative in their comments and behaviour, which can have painful consequences: irritation, sensitivity, complexes, and so on. However, if you let go of your preconceptions and mistrust, and focus instead on what people are really saying, more often than not you will find that their intentions are kind. You will realise that your sister is not judging your meticulously organised life, but rather that she admires your ability to seamlessly juggle your professional, family and social responsibilities. Similarly, your colleague does not see you as a sycophant, but envies the confidence you inspire in your boss, and your best friend is not criticising your classic outfits, but admires your elegance and simplicity.

It is up to you to look on the bright side and to listen to people when they compliment you. Instead of focusing on imagined criticism, pay attention to the people around you: your friends, family and colleagues are the best-placed people to see you as you really are. Learn to accept praise, hold onto compliments and acknowledge your good points. This does not mean being naïve (not every criticism or scathing comment is concealing a compliment!), but avoid letting your imagination run wild and give other people the benefit of the doubt.

Test: can you take a compliment?

How would you interpret the following sentences? Answer honestly and objectively.

- "You spend a lot of time at work."
  - You are overzealous.
  - You have an excellent work ethic.

- "Your naivety will get you into trouble."
  - You are easy to manipulate.
  - You inspire confidence in people and give unconditionally.

- "Your dress is clinging to you."
  - You have put on weight.
  - You know how to dress to accentuate your curves.

- "You have an interesting accent."
  - The way you talk is ridiculous.
  - The way you talk is charming.

- "You seem younger than you are."
  - You are immature.
  - You have a fresh, youthful face.

If you mainly chose the first option, you still have work to do. Reread the last section and take the time you need to start interpreting things, comments and people more positively. If you mainly chose the second option, well done! You have already made good progress and know how to take a compliment. The more compliments you take on board, the more able you will be to recognise and emphasise your good points.

Stand up for yourself

Not letting your insecurities rule your life is an essential step, but it is not enough: you need to overcome your self-consciousness to the point that you do not feel the need to hide your perceived weaknesses in public. The more you practice, the more quickly your anxiety will disappear. No matter whether your accent in a foreign language is very thick, your shyness makes you stutter or you are afraid of saying something stupid, ignore your fear and speak anyway. If it will reassure you, you could tell the other person that you are shy or anxious. They will then know that you are doing your best and will be able to help you if you stumble over a word. You can also laugh about your nerves with them – some gentle self-deprecation always helps to lighten the mood.

Broaden your areas of expertise

One excellent way of countering the effects of your insecurities is a healthy dose of self-confidence, and recognising and strengthening your good points is an essential part of this process. If you feel self-conscious about your level of intellect but have no desire to wade through lengthy tomes on history or economics, broaden your scope: find an area that interests you and learn about it until you are an expert. The amount you can learn is infinite: you just need to find your passion and let your curiosity do the rest. Read up on sports tactics, ocean currents or Aboriginal art, or take knitting, cookery or gardening classes. You will enjoy learning something new and feel that you are filling in the gaps in your knowledge.

Change your outlook

When our self-esteem is low, we tend to only see the bad in everything and our distorted, disparaging view of ourselves extends to a range of other areas. To silence your doubts about yourself, you will need to adopt a positive attitude, stop complaining and start looking on the bright side. Focus on all the good things around you and hold onto moments of joy. The more you take a positive view of the world, the more you will be able to see what other people like about you. You may even realise that something you saw as a flaw is actually a good thing, as it is the little things that give you your individuality and charm.

MAINTAINING YOUR NEWFOUND SELF-ESTEEM

With time and effort, you should now have learned to silence your doubts, recognise your good points and draw attention to your strengths. Now, you can start making the most of all that life has to offer.

Do not be afraid of letting other people form their own judgements and potentially criticising you. Not everyone is going to like you, and happiness and positivity will always attract jealousy. Let other people deal with their own issues and focus on yourself. Your insecurities have controlled your life and held you back for too long – now you need to make up for lost time! You have the rest of your life ahead of you, so get out there and have fun.

<u>**OVER TO YOU**</u>

You have set off on the right track by increasing your self-confidence, so there is no point stopping now! Overcoming your insecurities and managing to accept yourself as you are both good, but you can go further. Be ambitious: do not settle for simply accepting yourself, but learn to love yourself! Now that you are aware of your good points, work on developing them, and do not be afraid to draw attention to the things you like about yourself.

FAQS

ARE WE ALL EQUALLY SUSCEPTIBLE TO FEELING SELF-CONSCIOUS?

Yes and no. At some point in our lives, we have all felt self-conscious about one thing or another, whether it is to do with our physical appearance, work, surname or something else entirely. Occasional feelings of inferiority, unhappiness and low self-esteem affect us all. Although it is widely believed that women are more susceptible to low self-esteem than men, this is not the case: the problem affects men just as much as women, but may be less immediately visible. Everyone has compared themselves to other people and felt that they do not measure up, even the people who are seen as the most brilliant, attractive or powerful. Low self-esteem can affect anybody.

However, not everybody reacts to insecurities and self-consciousness in the same way, and we are not all equally well-prepared to combat them. Our experiences, our temperament and the people around us play an essential role in the way that we deal with our insecurities. Our attitudes vary depending on a range of factors and, contrary to popular belief, are not related to our alleged strength or weakness of character, but on our state of mind at a given moment.

For example, some people can disregard their self-consciousness at some points in their lives, but end up trapped in a vicious circle of putting themselves down during more difficult periods. Relatedly, some people lean heavily on other people for support, whereas others see this journey as largely personal. This range of reactions illustrates the differences between us, but this difference is only relative. If we feel overwhelmed by our insecurities, it is up to us to gather the tools we need to combat them: family and friends, a psychologist or psychoanalyst, motivation, determination, self-confidence and optimism.

ARE OUR INSECURITIES CAUSED BY THE MEDIA?

In spite of its far-reaching influence, the media does not, strictly speaking, cause insecurities. It strengthens, exploits and fuels them, but it does not create them, as they come from within the individual. However, it is undeniable that particular standards of beauty and success are depicted in the media every day and, above all, are presented as the only route to happiness, which serves to make things worse for people who are already vulnerable and suffering from low self-esteem. It is important not to put too much stock in the images presented by the media, as they are often fictional, retouched and staged, and do not resemble real life for anyone, so they should not be taken as a perfect model to strive towards.

ALTHOUGH I AM WELL INTO ADULTHOOD, MY MOTHER'S CRITICISMS STILL AFFECT ME. IS THIS NORMAL?

It is normal to be sensitive to comments from our loved ones, as these provide points of reference that give us a sense of structure. Our parents obviously play a major role in shaping who we are as people, but we need to know how to take a step back, as they are still only human and can make mistakes. Your mother's comments were no doubt well-intentioned, but she may not have realised that it hurts you when she feels the need to give her opinion on every single choice you make. It is time to cut the apron strings and stand up for yourself as an independent adult who is responsible for their own decisions. Explain to her that you would like her to keep her opinions to herself unless you ask for them, and make it clear that, now that she has raised you, it is time to stand on your own two feet. You can also control how you respond to her criticism: stay neutral when she makes hurtful comments and stand up for yourself. By acting like a strong, confident adult, you will show her that she does not need to worry about you.

IS PSYCHOANALYSIS NECESSARY TO IMPROVE MY SELF-ESTEEM?

Delving into the past to locate the source of your insecurities may be a good way of overcoming them. Psychoanalysis involves this kind of self-reflection, but it is a very personal, intimate method that does not suit everyone. Some people need to deal with their past in order to move forward, whereas others prefer to face up to the present.

The choice of a psychoanalyst is just as important, and maybe even more important, than the decision to try psychoanalysis. This is not a matter of asking other people who is good or bad, but of finding out who is right for you. You should feel safe around them and want to open up to them. If the first session leaves you feeling more confused than when you started, try another psychoanalyst until you find someone who gets you.

I HAVE TRIED EVERYTHING TO FEEL GOOD ABOUT MY BODY, BUT IT STILL DISGUSTS ME. IS COSMETIC SURGERY THE ONLY SOLUTION?

Contrary to what you may believe, cosmetic surgery is not a solution. The problem does not come from your body, but from the way you see it. If you have a distorted image of your body, no matter how much you change it, the image will remain distorted. You risk getting caught in a dangerous spiral, with endless operations that never leave you satisfied. Once you have got rid of your love handles, you will want bigger breasts, then higher cheekbones, then firmer buttocks, then fewer wrinkles, and so on. Your unhappiness does not come from your body, but from your mind. Instead of spending money going under the knife, spend time working on your psychological pain. It will certainly be harder to get results, but they will be more effective and longer-lasting.

I FEEL UNSOPHISTICATED COMPARED TO OTHER PEOPLE. HOW CAN I HIDE THIS FROM THEM?

Sophistication and intellect are both relative concepts. At school or university, we only learn a small slice of information, but all human knowledge has value. Even if you cannot name any Nobel Prize winners, identify Beethoven's fifth symphony or list all the elements in the periodic table off the top of your head, you can still be proud of what you know: you can work out the price of a sale item quicker than any calculator, you know everything about Robert Browning's life, you know all 2Pac's songs by heart, you are an incredible baker, and so on. Think about all the people who would love to have these talents, and focus on what you have rather than what you lack.

MY COLLEAGUES MAKE FUN OF MY LACK OF CHARACTER. HOW CAN I START STANDING UP FOR MYSELF?

We often associate character with being out-going, extroverted and expressive, so by extension we may assume that people who are less vocal about their opinions lack character. This means that your colleagues are wrongly taking your quietness for an inability to have opinions and stand up for them.

It is up to you to show them that they are mistaken. Even if your shyness stops you from loudly voicing your opinions, it should not be taken for meekness or submissiveness. Fortunately, there is no correlation between the volume at which an opinion is expressed and its correctness, so believe in yourself. Your opinion matters just as much as other people's, even if it is expressed more quietly. Taking the time to organise your ideas will allow you to speak clearly and concisely. There is no point forcing yourself to raise your voice; all you need is a calm, confident tone to win the respect of your colleagues. In no time at all, they will come to see you as a source of reason and wisdom in the office.

MY FRIENDS MAKE FUN OF MY LISP. HOW CAN I TELL THEM THAT I FIND THEIR JOKES HURTFUL?

No two people speak in exactly the same way. While some ways of talking are undeniably more unusual than others, this should not be considered a flaw. Quite the contrary: your lisp is a part of you, just like your killer smile and your sense of humour. If your friends tease you about it, they probably see it as part of your charm. If you still find their jokes hurtful, the best thing to do is to talk to them directly about it. They probably do not realise the impact their words are having on you. Tell them honestly that their teasing upsets you and that you would like them to talk less about your lisp. Do not forget that they have their own insecurities, even if they are less apparent to you. This means that they are sure to understand where you are coming from and will change their behaviour so that they do not hurt you.

We want to hear from you!
Leave a comment on your online library
and share your favourite books on social media!

FURTHER READING

BIBLIOGRAPHY

- Psycho Facile. (2012) *Complexes*. [Online]. [Accessed 30 October 2017]. Available from Internet Archive: <https://web.archive.org/web/20120426111807/http://www.psycho-facile.com/index.php?option=com_content&view=article&id=16&Itemid=30>

- Tolle, E. (2001) *The Power of Now: A Guide to Spiritual Enlightenment*. London: Hodder and Stoughton.

- (1997) *Trésor de la langue française*. Paris: CNRS/Gallimard.

ADDITIONAL SOURCES

- Ruiz, D. M. (1997) *The Four Agreements: A Practical Guide to Personal Freedom*. San Rafael, California: Amber-Allen Publishing, Inc.

- Tolle, E. (2003) *Stillness Speaks: A Guide to Spiritual Enlightenment*. Novato, California: New World Library.

- Tolle, E. (2002) *Practising the Power of Now: Meditations, Exercises and Core Teachings from*

The Power of Now. Novato, California: New World Library.

- 58 -

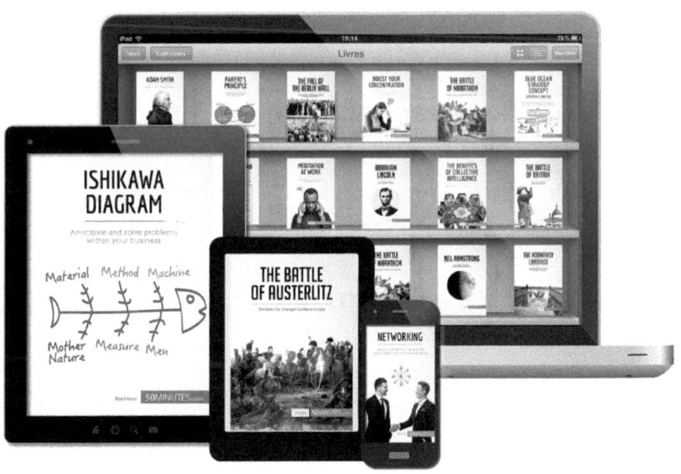